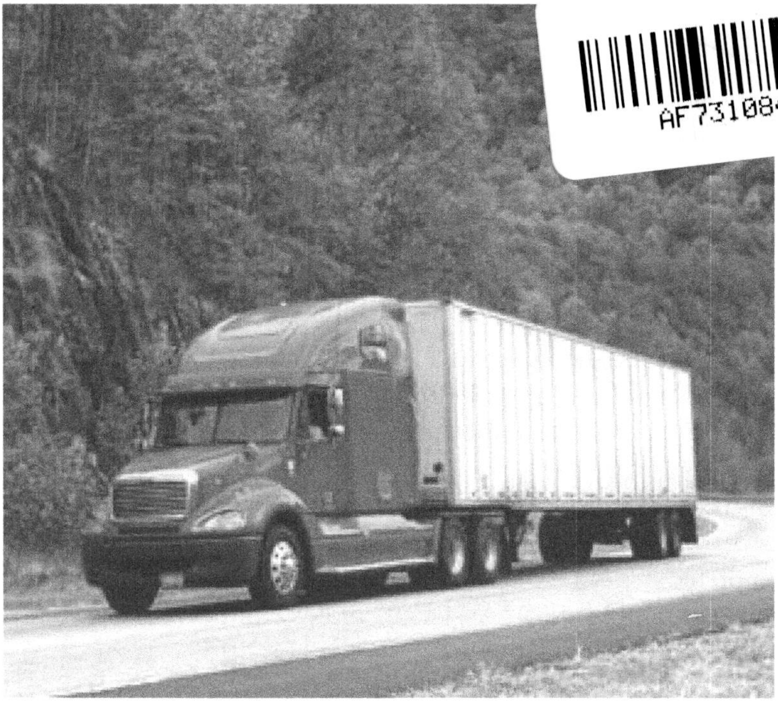

SIMPLY

PASS

YOUR CDL

PHYSICAL EXAM

T. Nikol West, B.A., PA-C, M.S., N.D.
Lauren N. West

About the Author

T. Nikol West is a certified Physician Assistant (PA-C). She has been a physician assistant and conducting CDL physicals since 1996, when she graduated from Kettering College of Medical Arts in Kettering, Ohio.

She continues to practice at a local hospital in Ohio, working in Occupational Health, performing CDL and Ohio Department of Education exams for CDL drivers.

She completed her under graduate education at Wright State University receiving her Bachelor degree in Psychology. She completed her N.D. degree in 2010. She completed her Masters of Science in Physician Assistant studies from PACE University in New York in December 2015.

She enjoys educating patients on how to improve their quality of life and prevent disease with diet and lifestyle changes that reduce the risk factors associated with many common diseases.

She currently lives on a farm in rural Ohio. When not working, she enjoys spending time with her children and farm animals. Her hobbies are fishing, boating, running, and the regular chores on the farm.

She is helping her daughter save and convert the family farm into a shelter for victims of domestic violence. The profits from this book will be used to improve the lives of those who are survivors of domestic violence and create laws to protect victims.

About the Co-author and Editor

Lauren West is a 19 year old college student at Wright State University in Dayton, Ohio. She is studying business and pre-law. She has encouraged her mother to leave an abusive marriage and complete this book to help her save their farm. Lauren is trying to raise funds to convert the family farm into a shelter for domestic violence victims.

The profits from this book will be used for domestic violence shelter and to raise money to help improve domestic violence laws to protect families. Part of the proceeds will be used to develop a safe house for victims of domestic violence.

Anticipated date of copyright/final publishing
09-12-18

Table of Contents

Simply PASS Your CDL Physical Exam

Introduction

This book is designed to equip commercial drivers, with the information needed to prepare them to pass their physical exam requirements for the Commercial Drivers License (CDL).

The federal requirements for providers doing CDL exams were changed in 2014, and there are now fewer qualified medical examiners. The examiners are required to be nationally tested and registered. In order for a provider to have a National Registry number they must have taken an approved Federal Motor Carrier Safety Administration (FMCSA) Medical Examiner Training Course and must have passed the National Registry of Certified Medical Examiners Exam. The information in this book is reflective of the requirements from the course.

The goals of the regulations are to ultimately protect and keep the drivers and the public safe on the roads. They are also to help to insure that the driver is not at risk of sudden death, or at an increased likelihood of disease or death.

My goal in writing this book is to help prepare drivers and the trucking companies, who hire drivers for the Commercial Driver License (CDL) examination. If the driver is prepared and brings proper documentation of current health conditions, he or she is more likely to pass the examination without delay in obtaining their examination certificate.

Having the proper information and being prepared for the examination can save the driver, and the company hiring the driver, time and money. If the driver is not prepared or does not have the proper documentation it may take days or even weeks to have a valid passing certificate. Failure to attain the examination certificate, may delay the driver from being hired or may prevent the driver from continuing to drive a commercial motor vehicle. If the driver allows their certificate to expire, they may be required to start the entire process of obtaining a commercial driver license over again. Such delays could prove to be quite costly due to time off, or possibly result in loss of employment.

The medical examiner's job to evaluate a driver's physical conditions and identify any condition or disease that may interfere with driving a commercial motor vehicle or pose a potential risk to the safety of the driver or the public on the roads.

This book is NOT meant to diagnose ANY condition. This book is NOT meant to treat ANY condition. It is important to work closely with the primary care provider and examining provider to assure that medical conditions are well controlled with medications that will not affect the driver's ability to safely operate a commercial vehicle.

The examiner will consider the following as potential risks when doing the exam:

-Symptoms of a medical condition or medication that may interfere with the driver's ability to safely drive or operate a commercial motor vehicle.

-Symptoms or conditions that may could interfere with the driver's ability to respond appropriately to circumstances while driving a commercial motor vehicle.

-Symptoms of any medical condition or any medication or medical treatment that could possibly interfere with the driver's problem solving skills or mental functioning in any way may affect the driver's ability to safely perform required tasks.

EXAMINATION FORMAT

At the time of the exam you will be expected to provide proper identification, including one government issued photo ID. Make sure you bring proper identification to avoid having to reschedule your exam.

You will need to fill out the history form with the required information:

-Make sure you know all of your medications or bring them with you. Know the reason you are taking each of your medications (what medical problem is each medication for). It is best to bring a list of medications with the dose and how many times they are taken in a day, and the medical condition or reason listed next to the name of the medication. Some family physician offices or pharmacies can print this list off for you from your medical records if you request a copy.

-Bring a list of any medications, foods, plants or animals that you may be allergic to and note the type of reaction you have had, and any treatment you have required for an adverse reaction.

-Bring the names, addresses, and phone numbers for ALL of your treating physicians. (If you have a cardiologist or other specialist physician make sure you have their contact information.)

-Bring a list of any surgeries or hospitalizations, including dates and reasons.

Preparation for exam:

-Two to three days prior to your exam avoid high fat, high sodium foods. Avoid all fast food, as most contain Monosodium Glutamate (MSG), which can raise the blood pressure even more than regular table salt. After your exam sea salt, mineral salt, Mrs. Dash or Himalayan sea salt are the preferred salt alternatives. Healthier choices at fast food restaurants are best such as: salads, lean meat such as turkey or chicken subs (remove top of sandwich and fold in half to decrease excess carbohydrates); baked or grilled lean meat options. Avoid: fried foods, extra sugars, soda pop and other processed junk foods.

-Avoid smoking or any nicotine products for a minimum of 24 hours prior to your exam.

-Avoid all products with caffeine for a minimum of 12 hours prior to the exam. Caffeine can raise the heart rate and blood pressure.

-Choose a whole food diet for a minimum of three days prior to your exam (A week would be even better). Include: raw fruits and vegetables; lean baked or grilled meat, eggs, and whole grains in appropriate serving sizes, usually ½ cup is a serving size for starches and grains; lean meats (3oz or a deck of card size is considered a serving size for meat) such as fish, chicken and turkey with no sodium or broth. Broth usually has MSG, which contains high amounts of sodium, which can increase blood pressure. Most prepackaged lunchmeat sold in the grocery store, is high in salt or may have nitrites or MSG. Eggs, beans and raw nuts are another protein option if you can eat them without the salt. The salt free nuts may be found in the baking section of the grocery store.

If you have any medical condition, including diabetes you will need to discuss dietary changes with your physician.

-A plate method diagram is included at the end of this book for those who do not have specific health conditions and are looking to improve their overall health. This is similar to the diabetic plate. This will be found at the end of the book.

-If you know when your exam is, and you can begin an exercise routine 3 months prior to your exam, that could help increase fitness, improve blood pressure, improve lung function, lower heart rate, and reduce weight, if needed. Walking in place in front of your TV during commercials, or walking around your truck 10 times each time you stop for fuel, may be a good place to start.

*****DO NOT begin any exercise plan **without** medical supervision and discussing your plans with your physician, especially if you have not been physically active, if you have ANY health conditions, or are on any medications.*****

-Avoid alcoholic beverages prior to the CDL exam. If the driver has diabetes, alcohol can raise the blood sugar. If the urine test shows sugar in the urine, this may delay certification. If the driver has an alcohol addiction or has been diagnosed with alcoholism the driver must discuss this with their primary care physician and report this to the medical examiner.

The following sections will give an outline of each body system examined. Each section will discuss common conditions and what the examiner may be looking for, along with what is required to pass the exam, citing specific guidelines. Specialist specific forms are included after each section when necessary. These forms may need to be completed by the specialist prior to the CDL exam to assist and expedite the examination process.

VISION

-The vision is required to be 20/40 in each eye tested separately by covering one eye at a time. The vision must also be 20/40 with both eyes tested together. The vision test CAN be done with glasses or contact lenses, but if the driver is tested with their glasses or contact lenses then the driver will be required to wear them at all times when driving.

-If the driver has not had their vision tested within a year and thinks that they may have had changes in vision since the last exam, it is a good idea to schedule an appointment with an optometrist prior to the next CDL exam. It is best to allow enough time prior to the exam to get new glasses or contacts if needed and get used to wearing them before the CDL exam. The amount of time needed to get new glasses or contact lenses may vary based on the provider, but allowing at least one month would be suggested.

-If the driver has diabetes, visual changes may occur more frequently, especially if blood sugar is not well controlled and kept in near normal range.

-If the driver has diabetes, an eye examination every year by an ophthalmologist or optometrist is required. It is best to bring a letter or copy of your exam notes from a recent vision exam to your CDL physical exam.

-If the driver knows their vision is not 20/40 or better, in each eye with or without corrective lenses, you will need to have an exam by an ophthalmologist or optometrist within the last 3 months prior to your CDL exam, and complete the Federal Vision Waiver packet. This can be obtained easily by searching online for "CDL Vision Waiver". The driver may also find it on: www.fmcsa.dot.gov. The CDL vision waiver process will be simple if the driver portion of the packet is filled out first, and then brought to the optometrist to complete their portion. A copy is then brought to the CDL exam.

The ophthalmologist or optometrist letter must:

-Provide a signed and dated verification on office letterhead.

-Include the type and cause of the lack of normal vision, including how long the driver had abnormal vision.

-Must state the vision deficiency (problem) is stable.

-Identify the visual acuity of each eye, corrected and uncorrected.

-Identify field of vision in both eyes and submits a formal perimetry test for each eye and interprets results.

-Identify the driver has the ability to recognize the colors of traffic signals.

-Verify that the driver has sufficient vision to operate a commercial motor vehicle.

***It may take 180 days for the vision waiver to be approved once the application is completed. It is wise to plan ahead so the driver's current certificate does not expire during this approval process.

IF a vision waiver is required, due to not meeting the 20/40 vision in EACH eye requirement, the driver must have a CDL physical exam and vision exam every year, even though the waiver is good for 2 years.

If there are known vision concerns, it is best to see an optometrist or ophthalmologist prior to the rest of the exam and have the eye specialist complete the vision section of the form.
The form can be printed from the FMCSA website:https://www.fmcsa.dot.gov/medical/driver-medical-requirements/driver-exemption-programs

HEARING

-The driver must be able to pass a whisper test at 5 feet distance or greater. This means that the examiner will stand at 5 feet or more from the driver and whisper words, letters, or numbers and ask the driver to repeat what is said. The examiner may also whisper questions and ask the driver to answer these questions to determine the driver's ability to hear.

-The driver's hearing may also be tested with a machine that tests for different levels of sound. The driver must have hearing loss of less than 40 decibels at 500Hz, 1000Hz, and 2000Hz in the BETTER ear WITH or WITHOUT hearing aide.

-If the driver passes WITH hearing aide he or she is required to WEAR the hearing aide at all times while driving, AND have an extra set of hearing aide batteries in the vehicle at all times, in case they are needed.

-Dizziness or vertigo is to be discussed along with hearing and vision if these symptoms are present. If dizziness is a symptom it is best for the driver to discuss it with the family physician and then have the dizziness thoroughly evaluated and treated BEFORE the driver goes for the CDL exam. There may be a 2-month symptom free wait period for certain conditions that cause dizziness. If the dizziness is caused by a medication, the driver's physician may need to adjust or change the medication to eliminate the symptom of dizziness.

-Certain conditions that cause dizziness may disqualify the driver, so it is best to have it evaluated as soon as symptoms occur.

CARDIOVASCULAR

The physician may ask questions regarding current cardiac symptoms. This may include questions about: chest pain, shortness of breath, heart palpitations or rapid heartbeat, syncope (passing out), ankle swelling, leg or calf pain with activity.

The driver may also be asked about previous history of heart attack, heart failure, heart surgery, vascular disease (blood vessel problems), aneurysm, or phlebitis (inflammation of veins).

It is important for the driver to know their medical history, including: the dates of treatment or surgery, the physician that treated the driver, address and phone number, or the hospital where the treatment or procedure was done. It is helpful to bring a list of tests or procedures that were done and any medications that were prescribed or recommended by the physician (including prescription and over the counter medications, such as aspirin).

If the driver has any side effects from the medication then he or she should mention them to provider. It would be best to discuss any side effects with the prescribing cardiologist and have those resolved prior to the date of the CDL exam.

It would be an advantage to write this information down or get records from the family physician prior to the exam and bring this information to the CDL exam. This will save time and help assure the CDL examiner has the information necessary for proper evaluation.

If the driver has a cardiac condition or has had any type of heart or blood vessel surgery, it is best to have a letter from the cardiologist listing:

-The medications the driver is taking.

-Verification that the driver's condition is stable.

-A list of the tests or procedures the driver has had, with the dates and test results. (EKG, stress test, echocardiogram)

-A notation of the next appointment or next date of testing with the cardiologist.

For a driver with a history of an abdominal aortic aneurysm the driver will need to provide the test results or statement to verify the size of the aneurysm.

-If the aneurysm is greater than 4cm and less than 5cm with no symptoms the driver may be certified for a year.

-If the aneurysm has to be repaired, there is a 3-month waiting period before the driver can be certified.

For a driver with an ICD/pacemaker (defibrillator): the recommendation is NOT to certify the driver to operate a commercial motor vehicle.

For a driver with a regular pacemaker: information is necessary documenting what condition required the need for the pacemaker. It is also advisable to have verification that the pacemaker is functioning properly, and the cardiologist does regular pacemaker checks.

For a driver with any cardiac arrhythmia (irregular heartbeat) it is important to have a letter written by a cardiologist that the irregular rhythm is treated and controlled. This will prevent the provider doing CDL exam from requiring a cardiologist to evaluate the driver in order to pass the exam.

A sample letter/form follows that may be filled out by a cardiologist and brought to your CDL examination.

CARDIOLOGIST FORM

DATE: ___________

I, ____
(cardiologist) verify that

____,
DOB: _____________ is my patient.

He/she has been diagnosed with the cardiac condition(s) of :

____

____

He/she has undergone the necessary cardiac tests:(FMCSA requires satisfactory ETT: every year for post CABG- beginning 5 years post surgery and LVEF greater than or equal to 40%; every 2 years for post MI patients, patients with angina- patient cannot have angina at rest; AAA must be less than 5cm) See FMCSA cardiovascular guidelines if questions.(www.fmcsa.org)

Check tests performed within the last 2 years:
___ EKG
___ Exercise tolerance test (ETT)
___ Echocardiogram
___ Other test:________________________

Please send copy of interpreted test results

This patient is taking the following medications for his/her cardiac condition and the patient has reported NO side effects that would affect the ability to safely

drive or operate a commercial motor vehicle.
Medications:

____

____

____

____

____

____

____

The tests results and or examination of this patient indicate that their cardiovascular status **IS STABLE** and he/she is in adequate cardiovascular status to safely drive or operate a commercial motor vehicle.
Next appointment or follow up: _________________

**If the driver has a pacemaker the patient is checked for proper function every ________ months. **

____

Date: __________
Physician Signature

____

____

Address/ Phone please print or stamp

CARDIOLOGIST FORM CONT.

OR

Complete if the driver is NOT stable

Date: ___________

I, _____________________________________
(cardiologist) verify that my patient

______________________________________,
DOB: ______________

He/ she is **NOT STABLE** from a cardiovascular standpoint and requires further testing on _______________ (date) or treatment before I can provide cardiac clearance to operate or drive a commercial motor vehicle.

________________________________Date: _______
Physician Signature

____

____
Address/ Phone please print or stamp

HYPERTENSION
(High blood pressure)

The FMCSA guidelines are:

Normal/Passing: Blood pressure less than or equal to 140/90
Stage 1: blood pressure reading 140/ 90 - 159/99
Stage 2: blood pressure reading 160/100- 179/109
Stage 3: blood pressure reading 180/110 or greater

Note: For untreated blood pressure greater than 140/90 and less than 180/110, a one time 3 month certificate may be issued. The driver must get treatment and have the blood pressure controlled at 140/90 or less at the 3-month follow up examination.

Note: For every 20mm of mercury systolic (top number of blood pressure) increase above normal blood pressure and for every 10mm of mercury diastolic increase, (bottom number of blood pressure) the mortality or death rate doubles.

*** It is important to KEEP your blood pressure well controlled.***

Factors that cause high blood pressure (hypertension) include: smoking, alcohol use, caffeine use, obesity, lack of exercise, increased age, high salt diet. Most fast foods are extremely high in salt and MSG (Monosodium glutamate). This is a good reason to AVOID fast food.

Most of the risks factors for high blood pressure can be

changed with effort. (Such as, stop smoking, reduce weight, increase physical activity, eat a lower salt diet- avoid fast food, and avoid alcohol and caffeine) The only risk factor that cannot be modified is age. This means that by: eating a healthier diet with more fruits and vegetables, getting adequate exercise, avoiding high salt, sugar and fatty diet, avoiding alcohol, proper sleep, reducing weight or maintaining your weight at a healthy BMI (Body Mass Index: based on weight to height ratio) and not smoking, a driver will reduce the risk of having hypertension.

To calculate your BMI, go to this link and it will help you determine a proper weight for your height.
http://www.nhlbi.nih.gov/health/educational/lose_wt/BMI/bmicalc.htm
It is important for a driver to avoid lifestyle choices that lead to hypertension, especially with a job that requires sitting and driving for extended periods of time. One of the most important health tips is to avoid unhealthy fast food while on the road. Walking and physical activity also decrease blood pressure.

Remember the choices you make today will affect your health in the future.

PULMONARY/RESPIRATORY

Questions the driver may be asked:

Do you have shortness of breath? Do you smoke? How long have you smoked? Do you have asthma, emphysema, or chronic bronchitis? Do you feel short of breath with activity or driving? Do you wheeze or have chest tightness? Do you snore at night?

If the driver smokes and is over the age of 35, the recommendation is that the driver gets a Spirometry/Pulmonary Function Test (PFT), to assure that breathing is not impaired. The reason for this recommendation is that adequate oxygen and breathing levels are necessary to perform tasks that require concentration and physically demanding tasks. Some drivers must throw tarps, straps, load, unload, connect or disconnect trailers, or other physically demanding activities.

This lung test is a simple test, usually done in the office. The test requires the patient to breath rapidly into a machine. It is best to avoid smoking 12-24 hours prior to this test.
If the driver has a normal PFT then they will likely pass this portion of the exam. If the driver has an abnormal test, then the driver may be referred to a pulmonologist (lung specialist) for further evaluation and possible treatment.

If the medical examiner hears abnormal lung sounds on exam, even if the driver does not smoke or has quit smoking, the driver may be required to have a PFT or schedule to see a pulmonologist (lung specialist).

Smoking cessation will help the driver to improve their health and decrease the risk of serious medical illnesses. Smoking contributes to cancer and heart disease as well as other medical illnesses.

There are many ways to quit smoking but the driver needs to find their reason that they want to quit first. The majority of people who successfully quit smoking report their method of quitting as, " I just made up my mind and quit."

One successful technique is to decrease by one cigarette per day. Writing the number or cigarettes for each day on a calendar will help to figure out the stop date. Start with the number you are currently smoking on day 1; then decrease by one cigarette per day until you are down to 3 cigarettes. Then, decrease to 3 cigarettes for 3 days, and then 2 for 2 days, then 1 cigarette and then stop date. It is best to start each day with the number of cigarettes for that day in your pack. Prepare the pack for the next day, the night before and put unused cigarettes in the refrigerator in a ziplock bag and those can be used for the next day.

Other methods include: nicotine patches, nicotine gum, chewing gum, chewing on a straw, electronic cigarettes, or smoking cessation medications or supplements.

For supplements:www.mynsp.com/manyajones

Each person is different and needs to find which method may work best for them.

Allergies

-For driver with allergic conditions: sedating antihistamines should not be taken within 12 hours of driving. Some allergy prescriptions and over the counter medicines can impair the ability to drive safely.
-Severe allergic conditions such as: uncontrolled sneezing fits, inability to keep eyes open, severe swelling or itching of eyes that affect vision, or medication that causes sedation are reasons a driver may not be certified to drive.
-If a driver has a life-threatening allergy (common causes are bee stings, peanuts, seafood), then the driver should carry an Epipen at all times in case of exposure to the allergen. An Epipen can be used in the case of emergency exposure to an allergen and can save the life of a person with a severe allergic reaction. A driver should go to their primary physician and obtain a prescription for an Epipen and get it filled. **Epipen needs to be stored in appropriate temperature between 59-86 degrees F. It would not be appropriate to leave it in the truck for extended periods of time at overly hot or cold temperatures.***

Asthma or COPD

-For a driver with asthma or COPD: if these lung conditions are well controlled with medication, it is important to have those necessary medications available in the commercial motor vehicle and store them properly so they remain effective.
-If these conditions are not well controlled and

symptoms of shortness of breath, wheezing, uncontrolled coughing or any symptom that could effect the driver's ability to drive. It is best to see a physician and get treatment so that the symptoms are well controlled prior to taking your CDL exam.

Chronic Obstructive Sleep Apnea

-For the driver with chronic obstructive sleep apnea (OSA): if a driver has sleep apnea he or she should bring documentation of their last appointment with the sleep specialist.
-It is important to have documentation of regular use of CPAP or BIPAP machine, if one is being used.
-Most machines record the amount of use of the machine each night and can print a record that will include an average of the hours the machine is being used. To be qualified to pass the physical the driver must show at least 70% compliance, which means using the machine properly 70% of days at least 4 hours/day.
-It is not safe to drive if driver has low oxygen at rest.
-If a driver is just starting to use a CPAP, there may be a wait period before the driver can be certified for driving. This means the driver needs to allow adequate time to get tested and set up for CPAP machine if necessary. This will allow enough time to document regular use of the machine.

-One of the main contributing factors for obstructive sleep apnea is obesity (BMI > 33). To reduce the risk, it is recommended to keep or work toward a body mass index (BMI) that is within a normal or overweight range. If the driver is muscular and lifts weights or does body building, they may fit into the obese category. It is up to the examiner to determine the "fit for duty" of anyone in this category. The extremely obese category is one that significantly increases the risk of obstructive sleep apnea, hypertension, heart disease, diabetes, stroke, cancer and many other disease processes. To check your BMI use the link: http://www.nhlbi.nih.gov/health/educational/lose_wt/BMI/bmicalc.htm. The driver may also find a BMI chart by searching online: "BMI Chart images male or female."

For most BMI Charts:	Normal BMI is	19-24
	Overweight is	25-29
	Obese is	30-39
	Extreme Obese is	40-42+

(no other category above 42 is currently designated)

-If the driver's weight is in the extreme obese category it is important to work with the physician to make dietary and exercise modifications to reduce weight and risk for diseases that can cause premature death. This extreme obese category previously referred to as morbid obesity because it will cause a condition that will end life prematurely.

-Other obstructive sleep apnea risk factors include: advancing age, large neck circumference greater than 17 inches in a male and 15 inches in a female, small jaw, and family history. The only risk factors that can be controlled or changed by a patient are obesity and large neck circumference. Proper diet and exercise may reduce these risk factors.

-Medical conditions that may increase risk of obstructive sleep apnea include: hypertension, hypothyroidism that has not been adequately treated, and Type II diabetes.

Sleep apnea recommendations from FMCSA expert panel:
http://www.fmcsa.dot.gov/sites/fmcsa.dot.gov/files/docs/Sleep-MEP-Panel-Recommendations-508.pdf

- The medical provider may ask the driver to complete a questionnaire regarding sleep. An example of the Berlin Questionnaire is provided at the end of the sleep apnea recommendations, which is located in the website above.

-If the provider believes that the driver is at high risk for sleep apnea, the driver may be required to have a sleep study or evaluation for sleep apnea before the driver can be certified to drive a commercial vehicle. It is important to maintain adequate health, which will reduce the chance of being required to have additional testing to pass the CDL exam.

Insomnia

Insomnia is a common condition that may be treated with medications that can help the driver to get to sleep. These types of medications have side effects that may alter the driver's ability to safely operate a commercial vehicle. These "sleep aids" take a long time to be eliminated from the body (long half life). These medications may disqualify the driver from passing the exam. It is best to have the physician prescribing these medications look up the half-life of the medication and the potential side effects along with FMCSA standards. http://www.fmcsa.dot.gov/sites/fmcsa.dot.gov/files/docs/Medical-Expert-Panel-Psychiatric-Psychiatric-MEP-Panel-Opin.pdf

It would be advisable to have the prescribing physician complete the form for sleep disorder and bring the signed form to the CDL physical exam.

PULMONOLOGIST/SLEEP SPECIALIST

DATE: __________

I, ________________________________, (sleep specialist/pulmonologist) verify that ____________________________________, DOB ; _______________, is my patient.

He/she has been diagnosed with the following condition(s):

____

_________________________, and was last seen in my office on: ____________________ (date).

This patient has undergone necessary pulmonary/ sleep testing:
(FMCSA recommendations: include FEV1 of greater than 65%, FVC greater than 65%, screening pulse ox greater than 92%, no hypoxemia at rest.)
(See FMCSA pulmonary requirements for more information)

______Sleep study
______Pulmonary function test
______ABG

Please send interpreted test results*

______Pulse Oximetry

This patient is taking the following medications for his/her pulmonary condition/sleep disorder and the patient has reported NO side effects that would affect the ability to safely operate or drive a commercial motor vehicle. Zolpidem (Ambien) and other medications with a similar half-life may disqualify the driver. Look up at

:
http://www.fmcsa.dot.gov/sites/fmcsa.dot.gov/files/docs/Medical-Expert-Panel-Psychiatric-Psychiatric-MEP-Panel-Opin.pdf

Medications:
____
____
____
____
____

The tests results and or examination of this patient indicate that their pulmonary status **IS STABLE** and he/she has adequate pulmonary function to safely operate or drive a commercial motor vehicle.
______ CPAP Usage is required by patient. Average nightly hours used ____________. Information obtained from machine record. (FMCSA recommendations of 70% of days at a minimum of 4 hours per day) Please send copy of usage record.

___________________________________ Date:______
Physician Signature

____
Address/ Phone please print or stamp

PULMONOLOGIST/SLEEP SPECIALIST

OR

Complete if driver is NOT stable

Date: ___________

I, ___________________________________
(pulmonologist/sleep specialist) verify that

____,
DOB:______________ is my patient.

He/she is **NOT STABLE** from a pulmonary standpoint and requires further testing _____________ (date) or treatment before I can provide clearance to operate or drive a commercial motor vehicle.

__________________________________Date:_______
Physician Signature

____

____
Address/ Phone please print or stamp

NEUROLGIC

If driver has a history of a stroke or TIA ("mini stroke"), embolic stroke, traumatic brain injury he/she will need an evaluation by a neurologist to be certified.

The neurologist may require tests such as a carotid doppler, EKG (a heart test that is usually done in the office), CT scan, blood tests, or other testing to determine the cause of the stroke or TIA.

Recommendations regarding stroke or TIA:
http://www.fmcsa.dot.gov/sites/fmcsa.dot.gov/files/docs/StrokeMEPPanelRecommendationsFINAL-508.pdf

Certain medications may disqualify driver: If the medication prescribed, has known side effects that may interfere with driving such as: reduced concentration, drowsiness, visual changes, or dizziness it may disqualify the driver. The physician will need to verify that the prescribed medications do not cause side effects that will interfere with the driver's ability to safely to operate a commercial motor vehicle.

The driver may need to have a letter from the prescribing physician to verify the driver is free of symptoms caused by the stroke or TIA.

A driver may **NOT** be certified if known epilepsy, dementia, seizure disorder (unless 10 years with no seizure and with no medications to prevent seizure), dizziness, vertigo, Meniere's disease, muscular dystrophy, or other similar neurological disorders.

NEUROLOGY SPECIALIST

DATE: ___________

I, _____________________________________,
(neurologist) verify that

_____________________________________,
DOB:_______________, is my patient.

He/she has been diagnosed with the following condition(s):

____
___________________________, and was last seen in my office on: ____________________. (date)

This patient has undergone necessary cardiovascular/neurological testing for their condition:

______Carotid doppler ______MRI/MRA
______ CT of head ______ EKG/
______ Echo
______Angiogram ______Labs

Please send copy of interpreted test results

This patient is taking the following medications for his/her neurological condition and the patient has reported NO side effects that would affect the ability to safely operate or drive a commercial motor vehicle. (Anti-seizure medications may be disqualifying regardless of condition it is used for. If driver has a seizure disorder - NOT qualified.)
Recommendations for stroke or TIA:
http://www.fmcsa.dot.gov/sites/fmcsa.dot.gov/files/docs/StrokeMEPPanelRecommendationsFINAL-508.pdf

Medications:

____

____

____

____

____

***IF the patient is on anticoagulation medication:
How long will anticoagulation be necessary?____________________________
How often is the patient being monitored if monitoring is required for the anticoagulation treatment?

____

The tests results and/or examination of this patient indicate that their neurological condition **IS STABLE** and he/she has adequate neurological capability to safely operate or drive a commercial motor vehicle.

___________________________________ Date:_______
Physician Signature

____

____

Address/ Phone please print or stamp

NEUROLOGY SPECIALIST

OR

Complete if driver is NOT stable

DATE: ___________

I, ___________________________________

(neurologist) verify that my patient

____________________________________,

DOB: ______________

He/she is **NOT STABLE** from a neurology standpoint and requires further testing on _______________ (date) or treatment before I can provide clearance to operate or drive a commercial motor vehicle.

___________________________________Date:______

Physician Signature

____

____

Address/ Phone please print or stamp

MUSCULOSKELETAL

Driver may NOT be certified if he/she has the loss of a foot, leg or arm. The driver may get a Skill Performance Evaluation (SPE) Certificate by an orthopedic physician or physiatrist if any musculoskeletal disorder is present that will affect the driver's ability to safely operate or control a commercial motor vehicle.

The forms for the Skill Performance Evaluation Certificate are available through the FMCSA at https://www.fmcsa.dot.gov/regulations/medical/skill-performance-evaluation-certificate-application-new-driver-application. The driver will need to carry the performance evaluation certificate in the commercial motor vehicle at all times.

For some musculoskeletal disorders, the driver may be required to perform a simulated driver's test to show they have the grip strength or physical ability to safely operate a commercial motor vehicle.

Some conditions, other than missing limb, that may affect a driver's ability to safely operate or control a commercial vehicle are:
-Osteoarthritis or rheumatoid arthritis
-Moderate to severe musculoskeletal pain or condition
-Previous spine surgery that causes pain or limited ability
-Deformities of body part, muscle weakness or atrophy
-Paralysis or decreased range of motion of a joint or body part.

These physical conditions will be evaluated by the medical examiner.

Some of the physical abilities the medical examiner will consider is that the driver will be able to:

- Grip steering wheel and have adequate hand strength for steering and shifting gears.

- Change tires, connect/disconnect chains or cords, cover loads with tarps, load or unload weight required by driver's company.

- Climb in and out of truck, climb, bend or crawl under or over parts of a commercial motor vehicle that may be required.

- Other tasks that the driver may be required specific to their company

Musculoskeletal pain including back pain, arthritis pain or other muscle pain must be controlled to a level that would not affect the drivers ability to safely operate a commercial vehicle.

Common medications used to treat pain or musculoskeletal conditions, such as narcotics, are **NOT** acceptable to drive a CMV. Non-steroidal anti-inflammatory medications (NSAIDS) that are purchased over the counter include ibuprofen (Motrin) or naproxen (Aleve) are usually acceptable. Common prescription NSAIDS include: Mobic, Celebrex and Arthrotec. These anti-inflammatories are acceptable medications to drive a CMV. Acetaminophen (Tylenol) is also an acceptable over the counter medication.

For questions about your pain medication get printed side effects from pharmacist and search FMCSA and "name of medication". General guidelines: http://www.fmcsa.dot.gov/faq/what-medications-disqualify-cmv-driver

DIABETES

A driver with diabetes who has controlled blood sugars **without the use of insulin** may be certified to drive a commercial vehicle.

The driver may not have sugar in their urine sample, which indicates uncontrolled diabetes. This is one of the reasons the urine is checked at the time of exam.

The driver may not have recently or currently been experiencing episodes of low blood sugar (which is called, hypoglycemia) where the low blood sugar results in fainting (loss of consciousness), seizure, impaired thinking or speaking, without warning. The driver may not have had an episode where the low blood sugar required the assistance of another person. This assistance would include falling or fainting and needing help up; or the driver's blood sugar being so low that someone had to get them some type of sugar to raise the blood sugar due to the driver being incapacitated or unable to help himself.

The driver must not have had a low blood sugar reaction within one year of the time of the exam or the driver must not have had two or more low blood sugar episodes, with symptoms described in previous paragraph above; with in the last five years.

The driver needs to have a diabetic treatment plan provided by their primary care physician and have regular monitoring of their blood sugar both at home (with a device that saves the readings or a hand written log of their blood sugar readings) and by physician office with labs. Physicians/providers usually monitor blood sugar every 3-4 months with a test called a hemoglobin A1C. This test provides a reading of the average of your blood sugar over the past 3 months.

Hemoglobin A1c test ranges:

Normal range:	4%-5.6%
Increased risk for diabetes:	5.7%-6.4%
Indicates diabetes:	6.5 or more
Goal for diabetic:	< 7.0

The driver may not be qualified if their diabetes is NOT controlled.

The higher the hemoglobin A1c, the higher the risks of developing complications of diabetes that may lead to disqualification for a CDL certificate. Complications that can be caused by **uncontrolled** diabetes are: visional loss; damage to heart and blood vessels-leading to heart attack, stoke, or damage to blood vessels in extremities; kidney damage-which at late stages can cause renal failure and requires dialysis; and nerve damage called neuropathy. Neuropathy can lead to abnormal sensation in feet or legs and possibly in the arms and hands. Neuropathy may cause a driver to be disqualified if it could impair the driver's ability to drive a commercial vehicle.

Some medications for diabetes may increase the risk of low blood sugar episodes, especially if driver skips meals or is not following a diabetic diet and monitoring their blood sugar appropriately. These medications that can cause low blood sugar reactions include combinations such as incretin mimetics, and sulfonurea.

The commonly prescribed brand names of some of these medications include: Victoza, Byetta, Bydureon. Patients on these pills (oral medications) may need to bring a statement from their physician stating: that they can tolerate the medication while driving a commercial vehicle, how often they are being monitored at home and in the office, a log of blood sugars taken at home and blood work from their physician. It is a good idea to bring a copy of the most recent blood work from the family physician that includes the hemoglobin A1c level. If the hemoglobin A1c is not below 7.0 it may be recommended for the driver to see a dietician and follow up with their physician.** form to follow**

The driver may not know what the physician doing their examination may require, so it would be a good idea to have the family physician fill out the form below if driver has diabetes (if not using insulin) in case a physician statement is required.

DIABETES FORM

DATE: ___________

I, ______________________________________,
(physician) verify that my patient is

______________________________________,
DOB: _______________

_____ He/she has been diagnosed with Type 2 diabetes.
The patient was seen last in my office on:

____________________.

This patient is monitored every ______ months.

Tests used for monitoring of Type 2 diabetes:

_____ Hemoglobin A1C every _____ months
_____ Fasting blood glucose
_____ Self monitoring glucometer
_____ Urine dip or urinalysis

Please send copy of any laboratory test results: **include Hgb A1C**

This patient is taking the following medications for his/her diabetes and the patient has reported **NO side effects** that would affect the ability of the patient to safely operate or drive a commercial motor vehicle.

_____ Patient is **NOT** an INSULIN requiring diabetic.

Medications:

____

____

____

____

____

*****IF the patient is on an incretin mimetic (Victoza, Byetta, Bydureon or other) a copy of a home blood sugar log and Hgb A1C must be attached.***

Next appointment or follow up: ________________

I verify that this patient **IS STABLE** and not showing on exam or reporting signs or symptoms that would affect their ability to safely operate or drive a commercial motor vehicle.

_________________________________ Date:______

Physician Signature

____

____

Address/ Phone please print or stamp

DIABETES FORM

OR
Complete if driver is NOT stable

DATE: _________

I, ____
(physician) verify my patient

____,
DOB: ______________

He/she is **NOT STABLE**, has uncontrolled diabetes, or is using insulin or requires further testing on ________________ (date) or treatment before I can provide clearance to operate or drive a commercial motor vehicle.

______________________________ Date:_________
Physician Signature

______________________________ _______________

____
Address/ Phone please print or stamp

A commercial driver who **requires the use of insulin** for diabetes must either:

1. Have a current Federal Diabetes Exemption form, **<u>OR</u>**

2. Apply for a diabetes exemption. www.fmcsa.dot.gov/documents/safetyprograms/Diabetes/diabetes-exemption-package.pdf . It may be easier to actually Google: FMCSA diabetes exemption application.

> The phone # to call for questions: 1-703-448-3094
>
> A Diabetes Exemption requires multiple steps that may take 2-3 months to complete. Start this process early enough to not have a lapse in your medical certification. If you know that your physician is considering insulin for your treatment start looking into this process and make necessary changes in diet, exercise and weight to avoid the need for insulin. It is very difficult to get the exemption.

The following are required to complete the diabetes exemption form and may take a significant amount of time to obtain all of the information required:

- Examination by certified medical examiner
- Examination by ophthalmologist
- Examination by endocrinologist
- Participate in annual diabetes education program **<u>OR</u>**

3. Have proof of your grandfathered status. This means

the driver must have the original letter from 1996 granting the right to continue to drive if they meet the physical requirements.

The driver must have both the Medical Examiner's Certificate and the FMCSA diabetes exemption and carry both while driving.
The Medical Examiner's Certificate may have a maximum of 1 year.
The diabetes exemption must be renewed every 2 years. It is best to start this 3 months before the expiration in case something in the process takes longer than expected.
The driver must have appointments with the endocrinologist, ophthalmologist, and diabetes education at least once a year.
The driver must provide a QUARTERLY evaluation checklist from endocrinologist.
The driver must monitor blood glucose using a device/monitor that records results for the physician to review or print them off so they can be reviewed at the time of examination.
The driver must record/check their glucose level before driving and every 2-4 hours while driving a commercial motor vehicle.
A driver who is recently diagnosed with diabetes (no prior treatment for diabetes) **and** requiring insulin must wait 2 months before being certified to drive a commercial motor vehicle even with the insulin exemption.
*** A driver who has had diabetes and is starting on insulin must wait 1 month before being certified and obtaining insulin exemption. ***

PSYCHOLOGICAL CONDITIONS

If you have been diagnosed with ANY psychological condition, including one that you may think is mild, such as anxiety, depression, "chemical imbalance", obsessive compulsive behavior or any other disorder, it is a good idea to have your physician complete the psychological form or similar letter and bring it to your CDL examination. A form is included at the end of this section.

Adult Attention Deficit Hyperactivity Disorder (ADHD)

The maximum time a driver with ADHD can be certified is one year.
A driver must follow the treatment plan set by their physician and tolerate the medication prescribed (or other treatment) without it interfering with their ability to safely operate a commercial motor vehicle.
The driver must have good judgment, have no difficulty with focusing attention, no suicidal behavior or thoughts, and no personality disorder and must not have inappropriate behaviors or psychosis.

Bipolar/ Mood Disorders/ Major Depressive episode

The driver must wait a minimum of 6 months to drive after being diagnosed and **must be symptom free for 6 months** after having a non-psychotic depression that was **not** accompanied by suicidal behavior.

The driver must wait a minimum of 1 year to drive after

being diagnosed and **must be symptom free for at least 1 year** after having a **severe** episode of depression, having made a suicide attempt or having a manic episode.

The driver must have good judgment and have no difficulty with focusing attention. The driver may not have any suicidal behavior or thoughts, and must have no personality disorder. The driver must not have any inappropriate behaviors or psychosis. The driver must comply with treatment set forth by their physician and any of the treatment or medication must have no side effects that would disqualify the driver or interfere with driving a commercial motor vehicle safely. It is a good idea to read the side effects of any medication prescribed and discuss any potential side effects with the family physician and pharmacist before the CDL examination. Some of these medications may cause a driver to not pass the examination. Remind them that you drive a commercial vehicle and are limited to those medications that will **not** affect your ability to drive.

Schizophrenia/Psychotic disorders

The driver must wait a minimum of 6 months to drive after brief reactive psychosis or schizophreniaform disorder diagnosis. The driver must be compliant with treatment and symptom free for a minimum of 6 months. The treatment or medication must have no side effects that would disqualify the driver or interfere with

driving a commercial motor vehicle (CMV) safely.
For any other psychotic disorder the driver must be symptom free for a year and the treatment or medication must have no side effects that would disqualify driver or interfere with safely driving a commercial motor vehicle.

Anxiolytic, Antidepressants and Sedative Hypnotic Medication

Hypnotic medication must be a type of medication that is short acting (with a half life less than five hours). Any hypnotic type of medication that is used must be prescribed at the lowest dose that is effective for the patient's condition.
The medication may be used on a **SHORT-term** basis meaning for a period of less than two weeks. To find out if your medication is acceptable, please check with the physician who prescribed it and obtain a list of side effects from your pharmacist prior to your CDL examination.
Anxiolytic and antidepressants must be non-sedating. Medications commonly used for anxiety can cause sedation and can affect the driver's ability to safely operate a CMV.

The commonly used type of medications that are less sedating are called serotonin reuptake inhibitors (SSRI's). You can look up the type of medication you are being prescribed by reading your package insert that is given with the medication by your pharmacy. The side effects of the medication you will likely tell you if the medication could cause dizziness, drowsiness, slow reflexes, affect ability to operate machinery, or other potentially dangerous effects for the driver. If possible, talk with the physician who prescribed the medication or the pharmacist who filled the prescription. These professionals will be able to tell you the potential side effects of the medication and whether or not it would be safe to operate a commercial vehicle while taking the medication.

These medications may or may not have any side effects that would disqualify a driver or interfere with safely driving a commercial motor vehicle.

If the driver is prescribed any of these medications, it is a good idea to have your physician complete the form for psychological conditions at the end of this section.

Another way to look up information is search online for: FMCSA guidelines on "the name of your medication."

A reference with half life of medications and suggestions from FMCSA expert medical panel can be accessed at: http://www.fmcsa.dot.gov/sites/fmcsa.dot.gov/files/docs/Medical-Expert-Panel-Psychiatric-Psychiatric-MEP-Panel-Opin.pdf.

Note some of these medications listed require 1-2 weeks of being off the medication **before driving a commercial vehicle. **Check this BEFORE your examination** to prevent being disqualified.

<u>Taking Lithium for psychological treatment</u>

The driver is required to have their blood drawn to monitor their lithium levels and the blood work levels need to be within therapeutic range or the range recommended by the driver's physician.
It is a good idea to have your physician complete the form for psychological conditions or provide a similar letter. You may also want to bring a copy of the most recent lab results from your physician's office with a lithium level showing it is in the proper range.

It is recommended that commercial motor vehicle drivers that take lithium be excluded from night driving since lithium can impair night vision and cognition.

The driver must be compliant with their medical treatment set forth by his or her prescribing physician and the treatment or medication must NOT have any side effects that would disqualify the driver or interfere with driving a commercial motor vehicle safely.

PSYCHOLOGICAL CONDITION FORM

DATE: __________

I, ____________________________________,
(physician/) verify that my patient
____________________________________ DOB:
____

He/She has been diagnosed with the following condition(s):
____
_______________________.

He/she was last seen in my office on:___________________. (date)

He/she is monitored by provider every ______ months.
Tests used for monitoring medication or condition include:
______ Lithium Level (**recommend limit to daylight driving only**)
______ Metabolic panel
______ Urinalysis/ Drug screen
______ BECK depression inventory or other scale

Please send copy of any applicable laboratory test results

This patient is taking the following medications for his/her psychological condition and the patient has reported NO side effects that would affect the ability of the patient to safely operate or drive a commercial vehicle. Benzodiazepines are NOT recommended for occasional or chronic use for CDL drivers. http://www.fmcsa.dot.gov/sites/fmcsa.dot.gov/files/docs/Medical-Expert-Panel-Psychiatric-Psychiatric-MEP-Panel-Opin.pdf

Medications:

____

____

____

____

____

I verify that this patient **IS STABLE** and not showing on exam or reporting signs or symptoms that would affect their ability to safely operate or drive a commercial motor vehicle.

__________________________________Date:________

Physician Signature

____

____

Address/ Phone please print or stamp

PSYCHOLOGICAL CONDITION FORM

1 OF 2

OR

Complete if driver is NOT stable

DATE: ___________

I, ____
(physician) verify that my patient
is____,
DOB: ______________.

He/she is **NOT STABLE,** has uncontrolled psychological condition, or is having side effects from medication or condition, or is on a medication that is not recommended to pass according to FMCSA standards, and would NOT be able to safely operate or drive a commercial vehicle at this time. The patient requires further testing on _____________ (date) or treatment before I can provide clearance to operate or drive a commercial motor vehicle.

__________________________________ Date:_______
Physician Signature

____

____
Address/ Phone please print or stamp

ALCOHOL AND DRUG ABUSE

Alcoholism

The driver cannot be currently diagnosed with the condition of alcoholism or alcohol abuse. The driver must have successfully completed a counseling or alcohol treatment/rehabilitation program if driver has been diagnosed or treated for alcoholism.
The driver will need to pass a drug and alcohol test, which is usually conducted at the physical exam location. The location may require an observed urine sample. This means someone may observe the driver obtain the urine.
The driver may not have any physical impairment (such as tremor, hallucinations, palpitations, seizures, delirium, uncontrolled hypertension or tachycardia) or side effect from the alcoholism or withdrawal symptoms that would disqualify the driver or interfere with the driver's ability to safely operate a commercial motor vehicle.
The driver must follow the DOT alcohol use/conduct guidelines.
Specific information pertaining to alcohol:
http://www.fmcsa.dot.gov/regulations/title49/section/392.5

***See additional guidelines at www.fmcsa.dot.gov.
*** Search alcohol and drug regulations.

Drug Abuse

The driver may not be currently using any controlled substances or habit-forming drug.
The driver must have successfully completed a counseling and/or treatment, or a rehabilitation program for previous drug use/abuse.
The driver may not have any physical impairment or side effect (including withdrawal effects from the drug) that would disqualify them from driving a commercial motor vehicle safely. Some symptoms of drug abuse/withdrawal may include: sedation, altered mental ability, slowed reaction time, slowed ability to think or process information, tremors, delirium, anxiety, agitation, headache, hallucinations or other symptoms.
The driver **may NOT** use methadone, amphetamines, narcotics, or marijuana, including marijuana for medical use.
Specific information regarding drug use:
http://www.fmcsa.dot.gov/faq/what-medications-disqualify-cmv-driver
http://www.fmcsa.dot.gov/faq/can-driver-be-qualified-if-taking-prescribed-medical-marijuana
http://www.fmcsa.dot.gov/faq/can-cmv-driver-be-disqualified-using-legally-prescribed-drug
http://www.ecfr.gov/cgi-bin/text-idx?SID=fb0b4afcff84aef52755d6dff7b8880d&node=se21.9.1308_111&rgn=div8

Resources

To look up how many carbohydrates are in foods download this booklet and it will be a great tool!
https://www.novomedlink.com/content/dam/novonordisk/novomedlink/resources/generaldocuments/CountingCarbandMeal_EG.pdf

The forms in this book may be copied and brought to the CDL physical exam if needed by the driver for particular conditions. The forms are to be used by the driver who purchased the book. Having the forms completed by the specialist prior to the exam will prevent delays in maintaining certification.

FMCSA = Federal Motor Carrier Safety Administration; SPE = Skill Performance Evaluation.

Adapted from Federal Motor Carrier Safety Administration. Medical advisory criteria for evaluation under 49 CFR Part 391.41. http://www.fmcsa.dot.gov/rules-regulations/rules-regulations/administration/medical.htm. Accessed August 2017.

Businesses may contact the author for consultations or driver education. Professional presentations may be scheduled in advance and are available onsite. Company discounts may be available for bulk orders.

Email : *passmycdl@yahoo.com*

Drivers requesting additional information on dietary or lifestyle changes may go to my website:

www.mynsp.com/manyajones

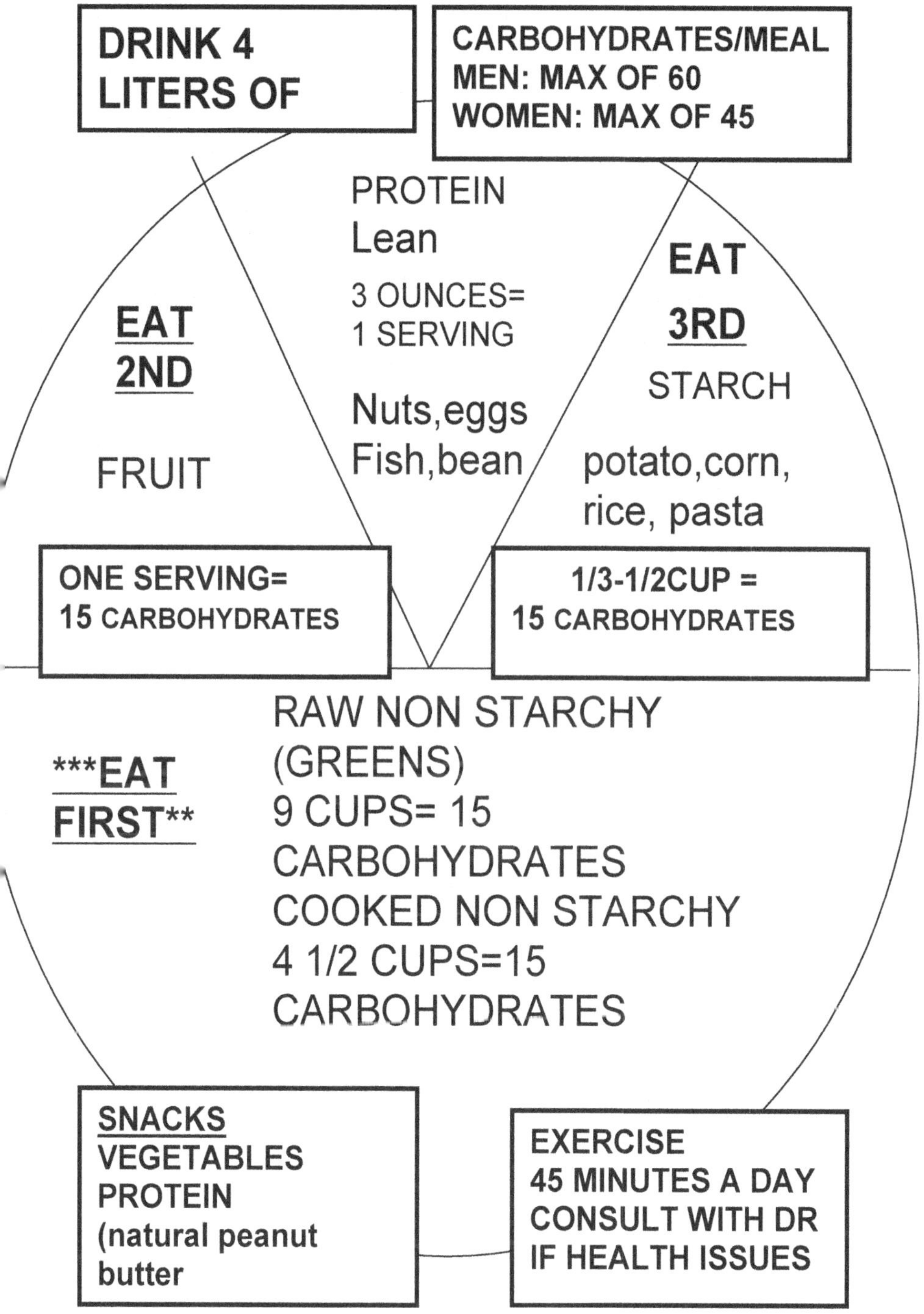
DRINK 4 LITERS OF
CARBOHYDRATES/MEAL
MEN: MAX OF 60
WOMEN: MAX OF 45
PROTEIN
Lean
3 OUNCES=
1 SERVING
Nuts,eggs
Fish,bean
EAT 2ND
FRUIT
ONE SERVING=
15 CARBOHYDRATES
EAT 3RD
STARCH
potato,corn,
rice, pasta
1/3-1/2CUP =
15 CARBOHYDRATES
***EAT FIRST**
RAW NON STARCHY
(GREENS)
9 CUPS= 15
CARBOHYDRATES
COOKED NON STARCHY
4 1/2 CUPS=15
CARBOHYDRATES
SNACKS
VEGETABLES
PROTEIN
(natural peanut
butter
EXERCISE
45 MINUTES A DAY
CONSULT WITH DR
IF HEALTH ISSUES

Made in the USA
Monee, IL
04 November 2026

67385923R10036